7 kinds of brain revolution success weight loss

Grace Tiffany Clark

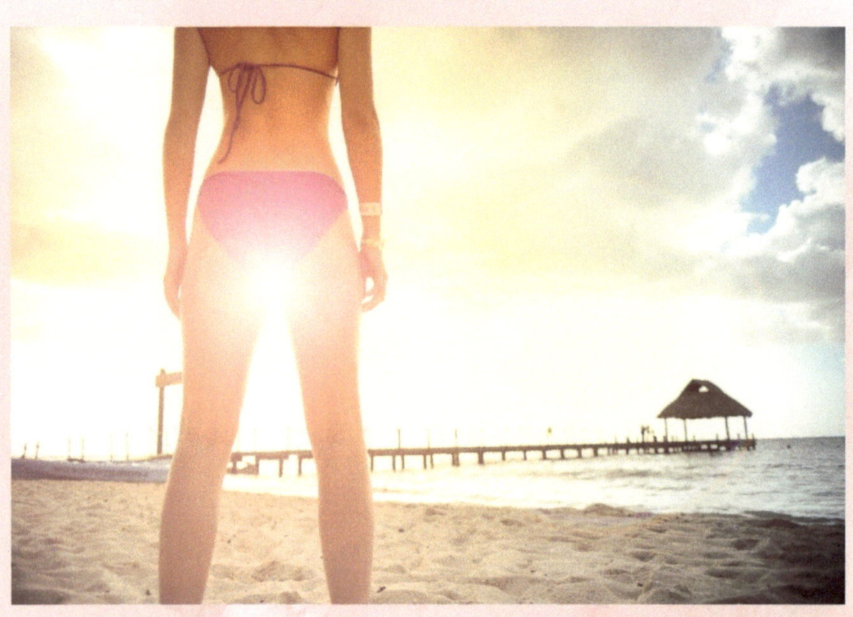

The significance of weight loss is to re-establish a healthy lifestyle. The key to its success is whether you do a "brain revolution" to fundamentally reconstruct the perception of food and lifestyle.

Table of Content

The significance of weight loss is to re-establish a healthy lifestyle. The key to its success is whether you do a "brain revolution" to fundamentally reconstruct the perception of food and lifestyle.

There are only two types of obesity, the first one is to eat a lot, the reason is not to cause obesity, and the other is to be weak, eat less, exercise more tired, body edema, the cause of obesity. Where are you? There are too many reasons for subdividing obesity, but we have studied in detail the type of food we eat, the type of food we eat, and how much we eat. You must first know which type of obese person you are and follow us. You can easily lose weight without losing weight

Chapter 1 Brain Revolution 1

The organs that control the weight are the heart, the heart is strong, and the body weight naturally drops.

Strong heart food recommendations

The organs that control weight are the heart, the heart is strong, and the weight naturally drops.

Section 1 Weight Loss Foods - 1. Minerals

The minerals needed by the human body can be classified into macro minerals and trace minerals according to the classification of the National Research Advisory Council of the US Department of Agriculture. The human body needs more than 100 mg daily, including calcium.). Chlorine, sodium, potassium, phosphorus, magnesium, and sulfur. The rest of the human body needs up to 100 mg daily, called rare minerals. (trace minerals).

Minerals participate in biochemical reactions such as enzyme activities, balance of body fluids, and energy replenishment of the human body. They play an important catalytic role. When the human body lacks sufficient minerals, it delays or destroys normal functions and eventually causes human gene mutations. , immune function and endocrine disorders, skin lesions, generate cancer cells and tumors, accelerate the symptoms of physical aging.

Mineral food sources • CalciuMvegetables • Magnesium: Nuts, Soybeans, and Cocoa • Sodium: table salt (sodium chloride, primary source), milk, spinach • Potassium: Legumes, All Grains, and Bananas • Chlorine: Salt is the main dietary source of chlorine • Sulfur: meat, eggs and beans • Iron: sesame, red meat, leafy vegetables Effectiveness of vitamins requires the participation of trace elements In promoting normal human biochemical reactions, the status of vitamins can't be ignored. Vitamins, also known as vitamins, include fat-soluble (A, D, E, K) and water-soluble (B, C, biotin, and folic acid) and more than 20 species, can maintain the normal function of the body system, help cells and protein metabolism, promote Bones and teeth grow, slowing down aging. Vitamins are macromolecular structures, most of which cannot be synthesized by the human body. They must be absorbed by food and vitamins must function. The key lies in whether or not microelements participate together. Vitamins are lacking. Biochemical reactions can still be achieved by relying on minerals, but they are missing. With minerals, vitamins will lose their effect.

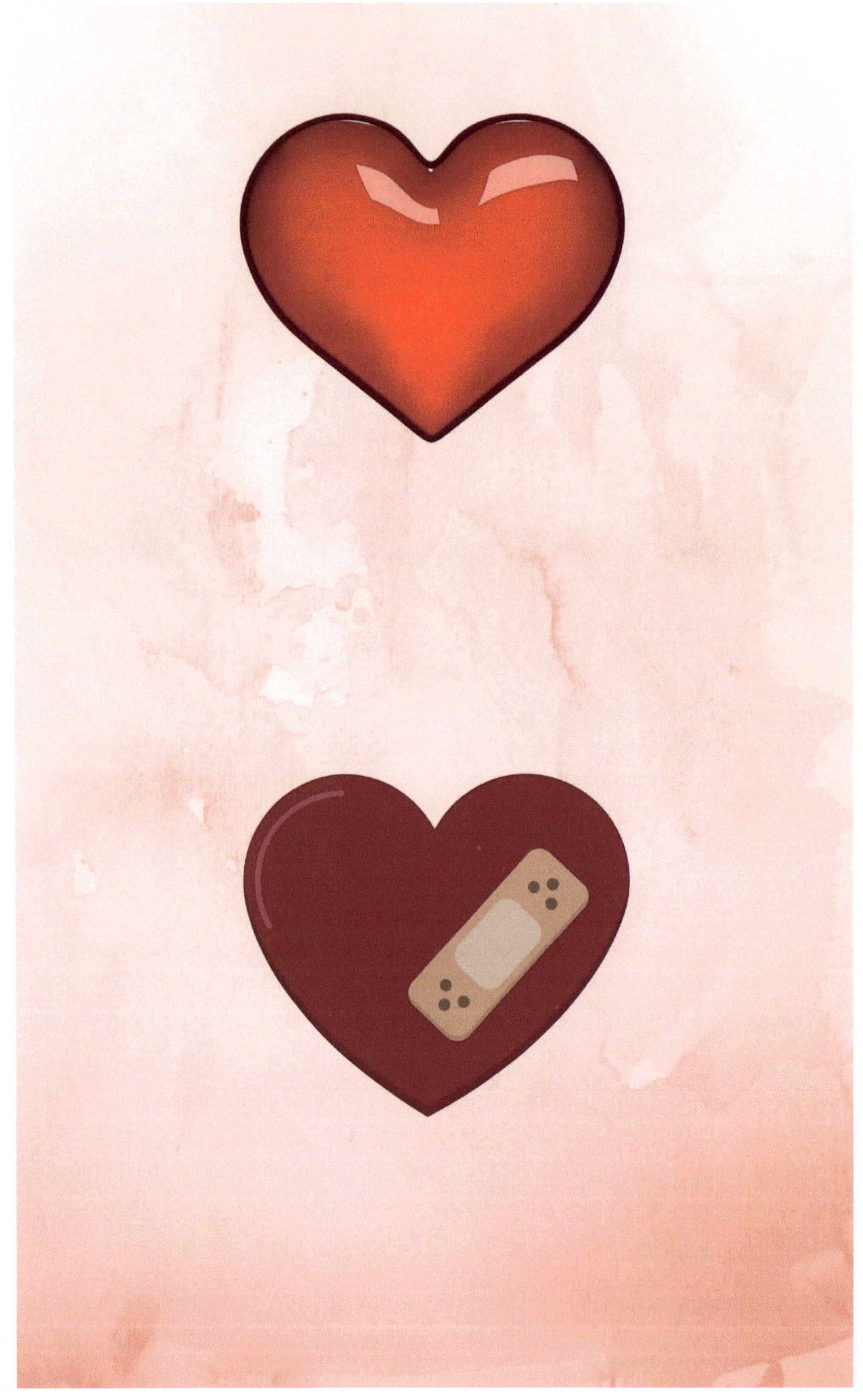

British scientist Joseph Black had discovered the existence of magnesium in 1775, but it was not until 1808 that another pure scientist, Sir Humphrey Davy, separated the pure magnesium. The source of magnesium was taken from the Greek place name Magnesia.

In addition to calcium and phosphorus, magnesium is the most abundant mineral in the human body, with approximately 21 g. More than half of magnesium is combined with calcium and phosphorus, magnesium phosphate, magnesium carbonate, and other magnesium salts are present in bones. The remaining magnesium is present in body fluids and soft tissues, and only 1% of magnesium is present in plasma. It is an ionic state and an important cation in cells.

Magnesium not only constitutes an important component of bones and teeth, but also affects almost all important functions of the human body, including metabolism, nucleic acid and protein synthesis. Therefore, it is also known as the "keeper of cell activity", from bone building to heartbeat to The conversion of blood sugar to energy is related to magnesium.

The main function

Promote heart and blood vessel health and prevent heart disease. Maintain normal muscle and nerve function. The combination of magnesium and calcium can stabilize nerves, ease emotions, and resist depression. Promote dental health. Prevent calcium deposition in the tissues and blood vessel walls and prevent kidney and gallstones. Lack of symptoms Neuroticism, trembling and shaking hands and feet. Palpitations, weakness, weakness. Kidney function is impaired. Myocardial calcification. Precautions Too much magnesium in the body will inhibit the central and peripheral nerves, resulting in muscle weakness, drowsiness, thirst, and so on, causing motor dysfunction. People who ingest large amounts of calcium and phosphorus or have impaired kidney function may suffer from side effects if they are taken in large quantities over a long period of time.

What food contains magnesium Animal foods: seafood, fish, meat, milk Plant foods: grains, wheat germ, figs, beans, almonds, stone fruits, dark green vegetables, bananas. Others: brewer's yeast.

Who should add?

Drinkers should pay attention to supplement magnesium. People who consume alcohol often have low levels of magnesium, so drinking alcohol increases the risk of heart disease and osteoporosis. Western diets generally have a lower magnesium content than the oriental diet. Most Americans are unable to obtain sufficient amounts of magnesium from foods, especially women who often lack magnesium. People who prefer Western diet must pay attention to magnesium intake. Women who use contraceptives or take estrus hormones must consume large amounts of magnesium. Expert advice Magnesium can help fat burn and generate energy, which is equally important for men and women. If you are always feeling tired and gradually gain weight, it may be a sign of magnesium deficiency. Post-menopausal women are particularly prone to magnesium deficiency, so blood clotting often occurs, leading to heart disease and stroke. In addition to the lack of magnesium in the body in addition to easy to increase heart disease in women, but also cause another problem, that is,

osteoporosis Intimate tips: During weight loss, it is best to eat minerals containing magnesium fruit, my advice is apple, why is apple, on the one hand is easy to obtain, on the one hand is apple's high magnesium content, eat apples in addition to weight loss, also Will make you feel good.

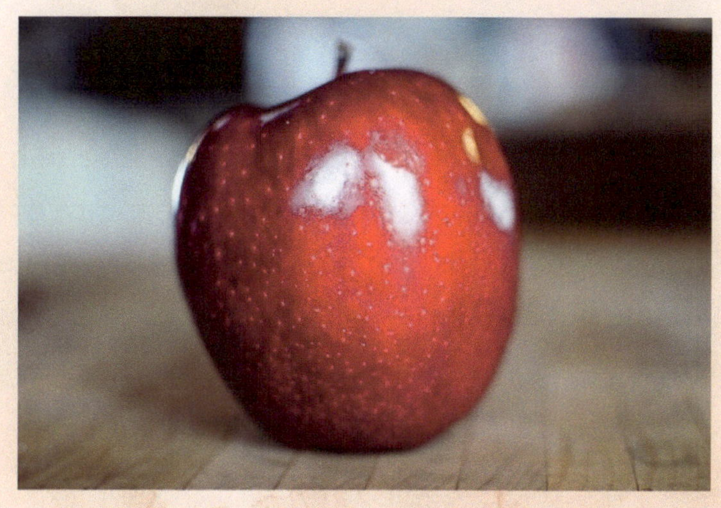

apple's high magnesium content, eat apples in addition to weight loss, also Will make you feel good.

Chapter 2 Brain Revolution 2.

Ingest whole food

The suggestion of protein should be followed with the idea of bringing forward a revolution in the brain to try to eat the original appearance of the food. It is natural. Do not eat processed foods, such as meat, but you can eat beef, pork, chicken, fish, etc. but do not eat sausage, bacon. Meat, or processed meatballs, fish balls, canned food.

Section 1 Weight Loss Foods - Intake of Enough Protein The first aspect:

The reaction of blood glucose, compared to starchy foods, the speed of protein digestion is much slower, his effect on blood sugar is slowly rising, and can even delay the speed of food digestion, with the function of stabilizing blood sugar, And it allows the blood sugar to reach a high level, also makes the brain have a considerable degree of pleasure, more importantly, so that the stability of blood sugar can make this sense of pleasure and satiety, lasting four to five hours until the next meal is normal Eating.

Secondly, during the weight loss period, our physiological function changes, and it will preferentially decompose protein as an energy source and cause the loss of muscles. If we do not take enough protein, the muscles that decrease will be much more than fat during weight loss. Weight loss, but body fat rate increases, has a negative impact on health, and will reduce the basal metabolic rate, forming a so-called easy fat physique, so it is even more difficult to want to use food to control weight programs Achieved, a little carelessness, resumption of fat, after the resumption of fat, fat and muscle ratio is even more disparity, making it more difficult to reduce weight next time.

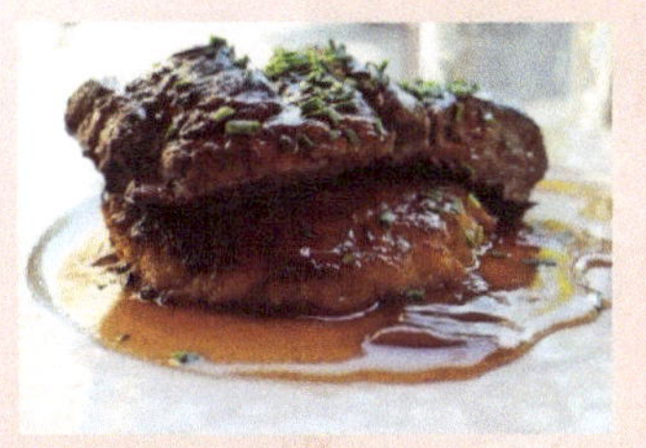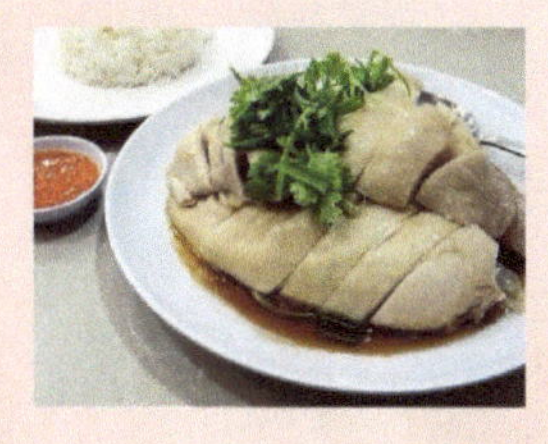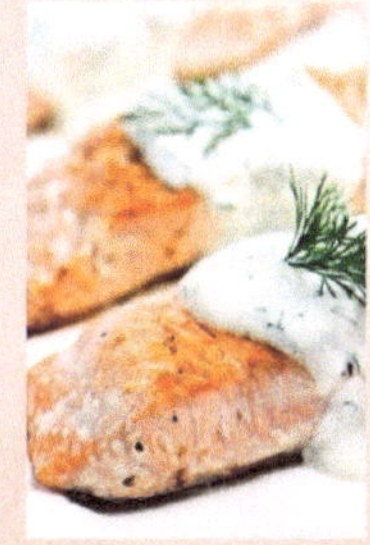

GOOD TO EAT NATURE FOODS

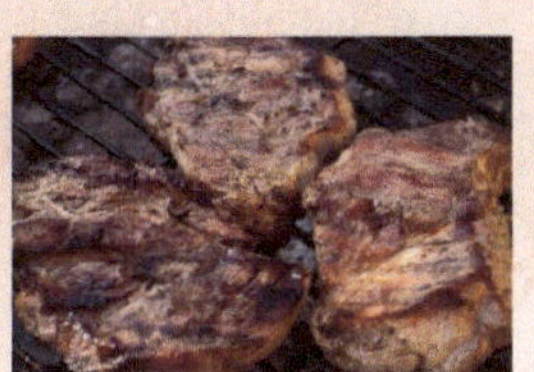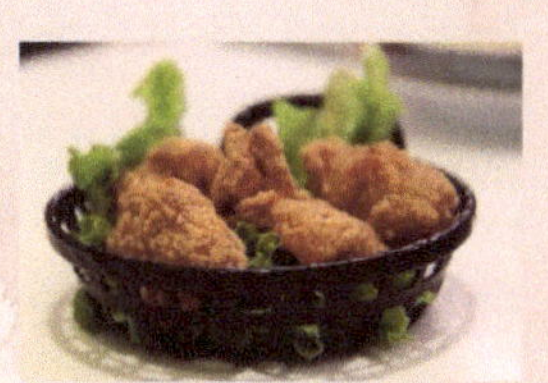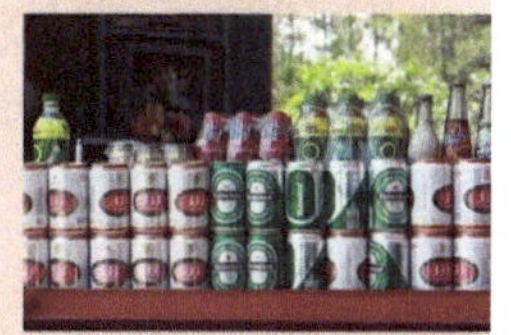

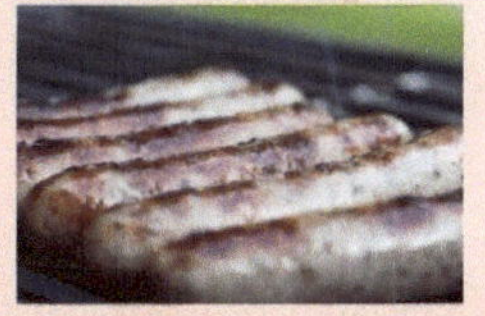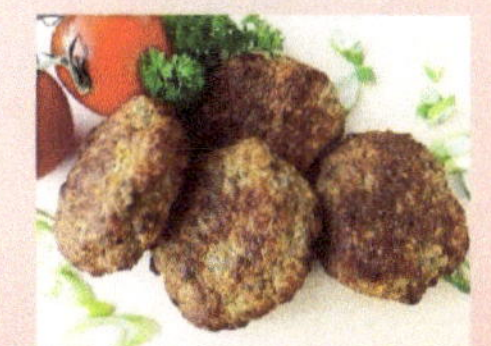

DON'T EAT THESE NOT NATURE FOODS

Chapter 3 Brain Revolution 3

Treat fruits correctly

Section 1 The fruit is too sweet to replace the dinner and vegetables

The idea of fruit in the average person seems to be a low-calorie healthy food. Nutrition experts and doctors often recommend that you eat more fruit, but the average weight of fruits and vegetables is about two to three times higher than the average weight of fruits. Fructose is very easily absorbed and converted into triglyceride to form fats. Therefore, in the course of weight loss, the amount of fruit must be taken in an appropriate amount. Fruits must not be used in place of vegetables, and some vegetables themselves are fruit and vegetables such as tomatoes and cucumbers. Apples, etc., These fruits and vegetables contain fruit-like nutrients, but there is no adverse reaction caused by too much fructose and are usually very convenient to prepare, they should eat more.   Fruits in addition to fructose, dietary fiber, number of phytochemicals, vitamins, beauty skin, good health, anti-aging, very helpful. Water-soluble dietary fiber can also delay gastric emptying time, to avoid severe fluctuations in blood sugar, cause Obesity, fruits have many benefits, but can't be a dinner, fruit is not like protein, fat foods stay longer in the body, if you only eat fruit when you eat dinner for more than an hour, you will be hungry, but will eat indiscriminately Fat.

How to eat fruit in the second quarter?

1. Attention to fruit calories: The highest calorie fruit is durian, banana, custard apple.

2. Choose low-glycemic index fruit: Although the fruit is sweet, but her dietary fiber is high, it still belongs to the low-glycemic index

Low-glycemic index fruit: kiwi, small tomatoes, guava, apples, oranges, cherries, eat more

Fruits in the Sugar Index: grapes, pineapples, papaya, strawberries, mangoes, bananas. Don't eat too much.

High-glycemic index fruit: durian, watermelon, eat less.

3. Variety, change, not excessive, one day the amount of fruit is probably about one to two bowls of rice, because the fruit has a lot of dietary fiber, if you want to eat do not labeled fruit juice, filter out the residue, if you filter out the residue, instead Loss of dietary fiber, causing blood sugar to rise, causing obesity.

4. How to eat fruit during weight loss? To pick low-calorie and low-glycemic index fruit, happy to eat fruit, not afraid of getting fat.

Low-glycemic index

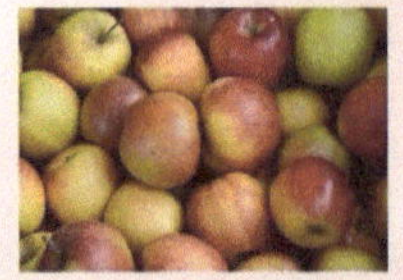 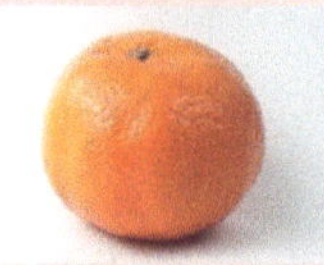 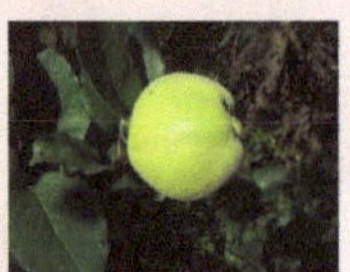

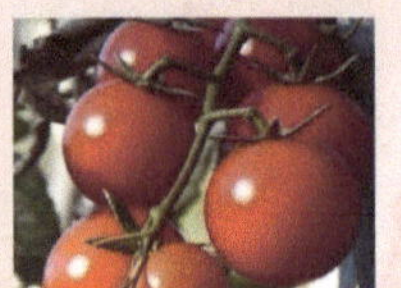 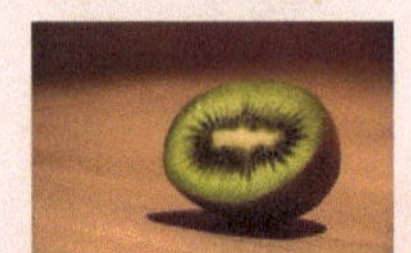 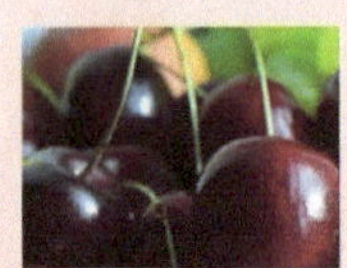

Fruits in the Sugar Index:

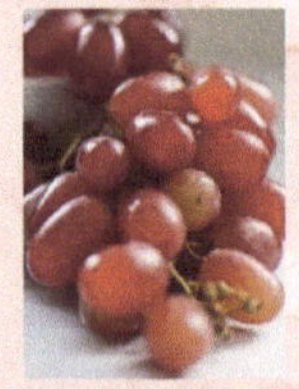 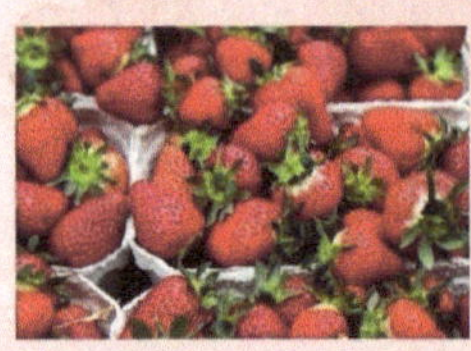 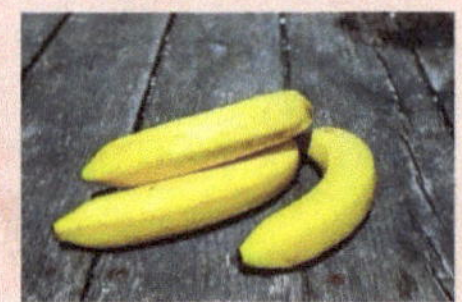

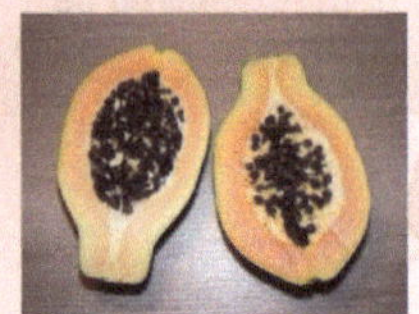 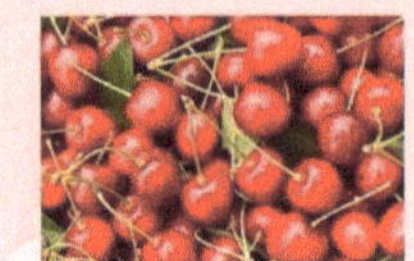 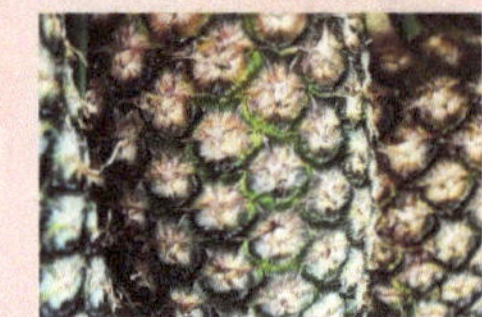

High-glycemic index

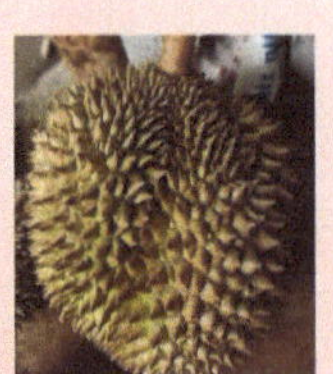 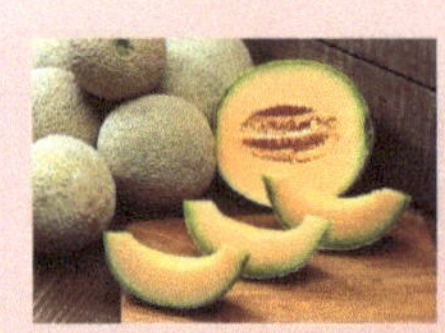 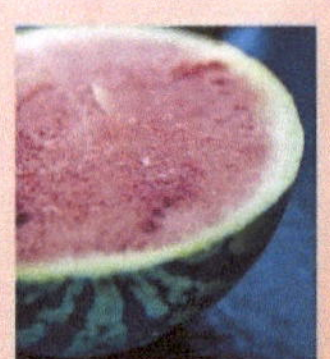

Chapter 4 Brain Revolution 4

Proportion of weight loss food

So, in addition to strengthening minerals, adequate protein, and how much starch is consumed, weight-reducing foods have a good weight loss ratio. In 2011 Harvard University School of Public Security based on their years of research on obesity and nutrition literature, put forward the concept of "healthy diet plate", 50% fruits and vegetables, 25% starch, 25% protein, and my side

The suggestion is that **50% of vegetables should be raised to 35% and starch to 15%.**

 The effect of weight loss will be even better. Why to reduce carbohydrates is mainly to balance blood sugar, avoid lower blood sugar, and cause hunger. Too much food, enough protein, but also the main source of muscle production.

Proportion of weight loss food

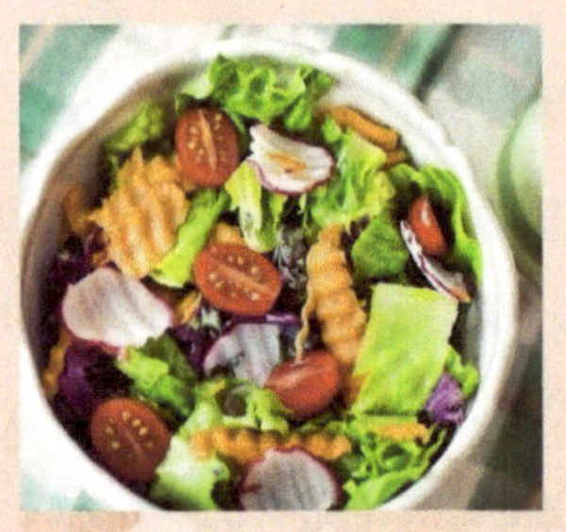 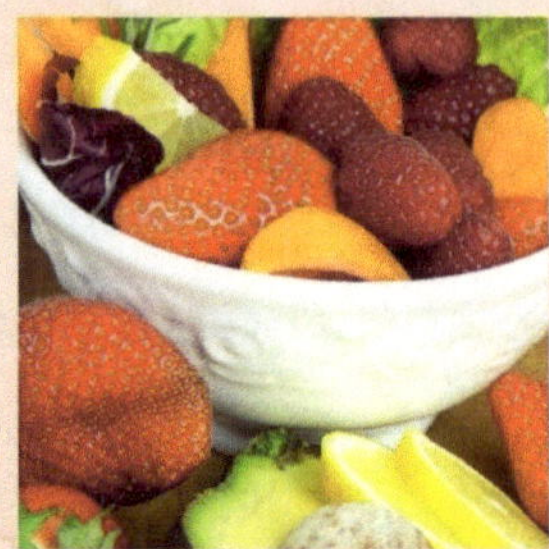

50% fruits and vegetables

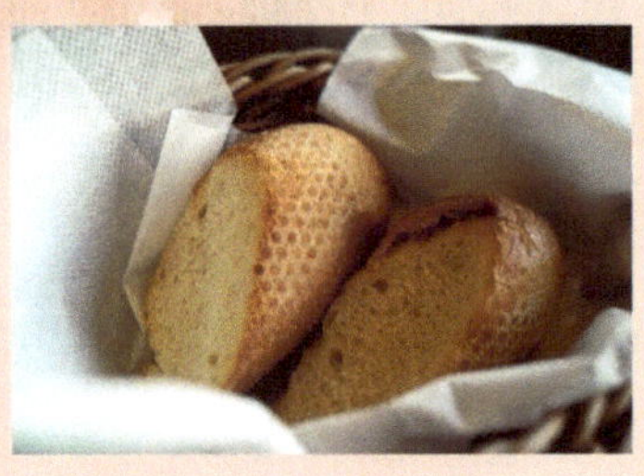 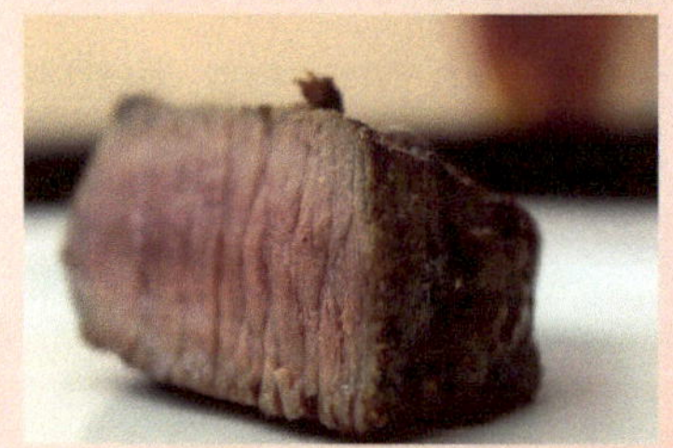

15% Starch   35% Protein

Chapter 5 Brain Revolution 5

The amount of exercise changes, weight will change

Can exercise help to lose weight?

 Of course, yes. Exercise can make you besides getting thinner, but also make you more beautiful and strong, but I am a lazy person. What kind of exercise do I have to do? How much time do I have to exercise each day? Let's make my body look better? Here we need a "brain revolution"

In the first quarter, why did you exercise and your body weight did not move?

1. It is recommended that the amount of exercise be changed, the body weight will change, and the body will not be comfortable. The body weight can effectively change the weight and achieve successful weight loss.

 2. It is impossible to see the effects of weight loss in a short period of time. It is only possible to integrate exercise into life.

 3. The first scenario: Unbalanced movements: People who do not exercise normally, drive cars when they go out, do not want to go one step at a time, do a lot of climbing and exercise on holiday, because you suddenly exercise a lot and the body produces a lot of energy. In a sudden situation, the metabolism of the body will slow down. The second situation: weak people, weak people have a weak heart, metabolism is slow, not suitable for intense sports.

How to choose the right sport in the second quarter The best sport is aerobic exercise.

The most effective aerobic exercise is to reach 120 beats, walk 45 minutes, or walk 6 kilometers.

2. Many people do aerobic exercise, go for a walk, and run. If you are not skinny because the body has adapted to your regular exercise, the exercise should not be deliberate, as long as it continues and integrates into your life.

3. It is recommended that the amount of exercise be changed, the body weight will change, and the body will not be comfortable in order to effectively change the weight and achieve successful weight loss.

4. Way: In the first week, exercise once (about 45 minutes each time).
In the second week, exercise is two times
The third week, exercise three times
The fourth week, exercise four times
Take a rest for two weeks and return.
The first week, the exercise begins once.

5. Intimate tips: We don't just suggest changes in the way of exercise but also provide a new idea. It is recommended to "massage the waist." Most people who are obese usually have more fat around their waist, which means poor blood circulation and inability to provide nutrients. Provide, if you can add a massage waist, and you are very convenient to do, can also be done in the office, will greatly help the weight loss process.

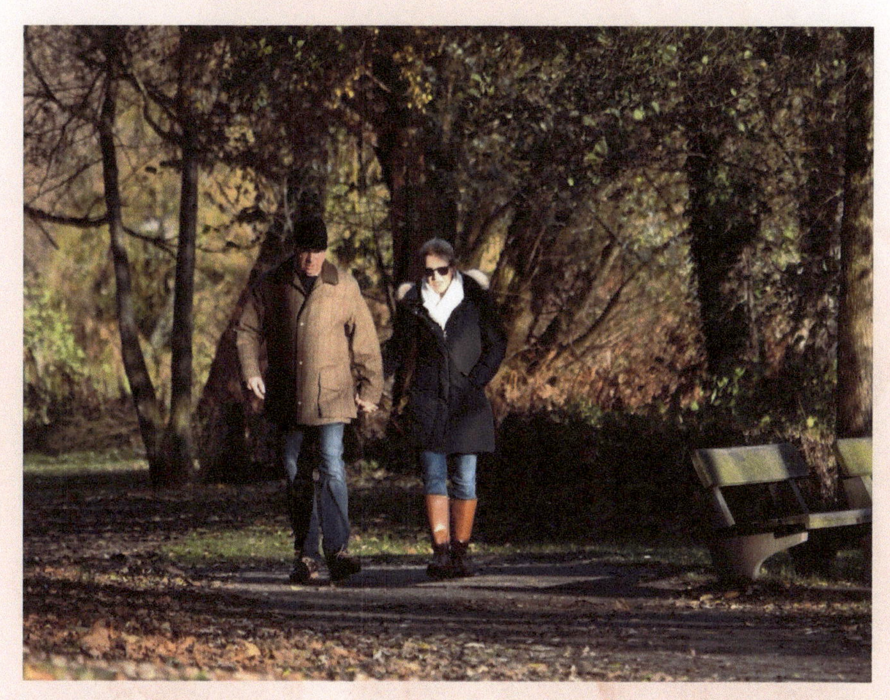

The most effective aerobic exercise is to reach 120 beats, walk 45 minutes,

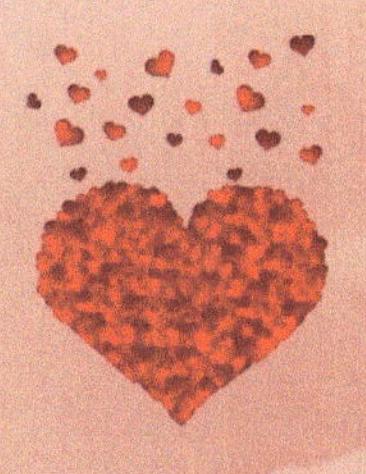

Chapter 6 Brain Revolution 6

How to drink and drink during weight loss?

Section 1 How much water do normal people drink each day?

Any nutrients enter the body and waste is discharged from the body, but they must be transported by water. However, if you are losing weight, you must be able to drink or drink a lot of water. It feels very contradictory. Normally, we should drink the amount we need in one day. Normal For example, the amount of water an adult drinks each day is about 30 times that of a body weight. For example, if a person weighs 50 kg, the amount of water consumed on that day is about 1,500 cc.

Section 2 How much water to drink during weight loss?

If you are losing weight. You need to drink about 50 times of your body weight every day, that is, 2500cc. Before exercise, during and after exercise, you have to replenish plenty of water. When you drink too little water, your body will think that it will encounter drought and it will start the mechanism of water storage. Keep water in the body as much as possible, so you do not drink enough water, which will cause the body's edema, the type of drink, as long as no sugar, no ice liquid, boiled water is the best choice

If it is coffee and tea, it cannot be calculated in the amount of water in a day. Drink more during the day and a little less at night to avoid affecting sleep. Drink water can't drink too much at any one time. Drink about 200cc for about half an hour and drink too fast. If you drink more than 1000cc in one hour, it is easy to cause hyponatremia, which is water poisoning. If you drink water and you want to go to the toilet in ten minutes, you are still thirsty, or you need to add electrolytes after losing a lot of water.

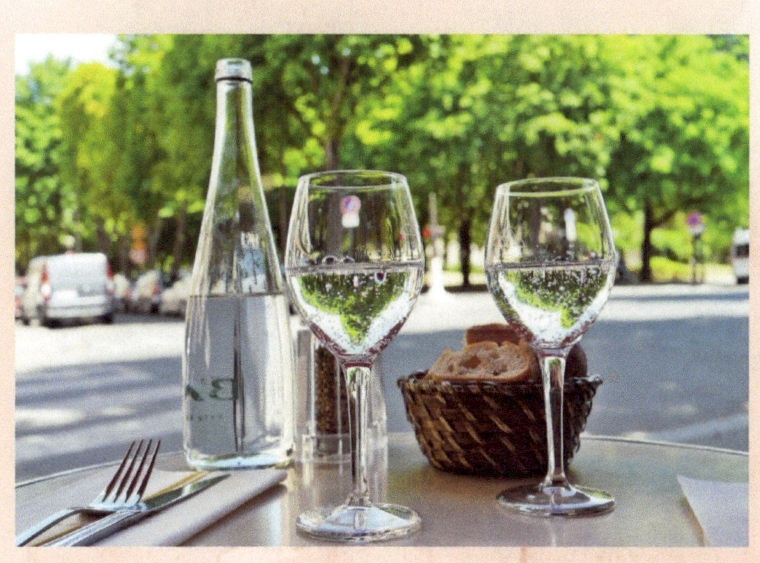

If you are losing weight. You need to drink about 50 times of your body weight every day,

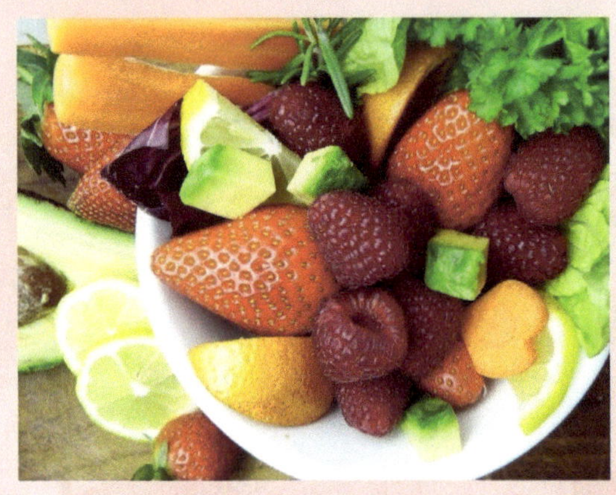

good to eat

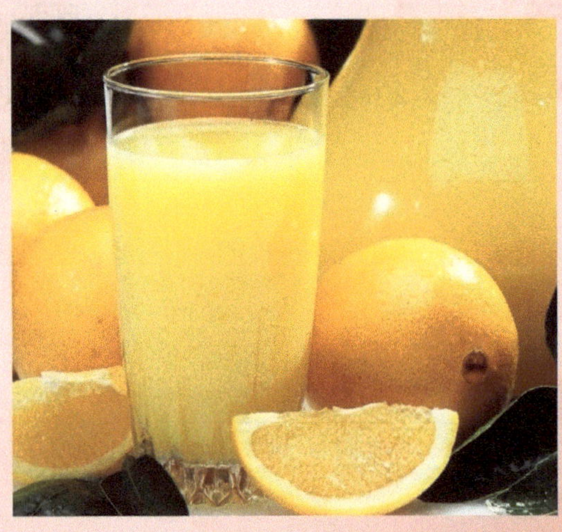

juice no good

Chapter 7 Brain Revolution 7

What happens to weight stagnation during weight loss?

Weight loss during weight loss will not fall like a slide, but will be like a ladder, weight loss period Many people lose weight for a period of time. When they experience a period of stagnation, how do they work hard and do not move their body weight?

There are two reasons for stagnation in the first quarter:

1. The first reason is that the physical protection mechanism affects: As the body weight is reduced to 10% of the body weight, it will encounter a stagnation period and start a mechanism to protect the body, because the body will think that it has encountered some disaster, and in order to protect the body, and start protection Physical mechanism, maintain weight, the body will think of ways to resist, and adjust the metabolic mechanism, then the weight will not move.

2. To eat less, you must eat more. If you have a lot of exercise, you will reduce the exercise and say nothing to your body. When the body believes, metabolism will naturally recover.

3. The second reason is that the body adapts. The Harvard nutritionist puts forward a set-point theory: the body will set a target weight according to the diet and lifestyle. This is the set point. For example, I changed from three meals a day to four meals a day. It will change from the set point from 65kg to 67kg. After a certain period of time, the body will adapt and the metabolism will stagnate.

4. Solution: How to break the balance and lower the set point:
 A healthy and positive approach is to increase the intensity of exercise, disrupt the balance, and make the body feel change. The set point will be lowered. Another negative method is to reduce the amount of food. , break the balance, but this must be during weight loss, normal diet, this is a fierce diet, so during weight loss, you can't start

with intense diet, so that the body will not receive any changes, if used in this can instead change body weight.

5. Weight loss during weight loss will not fall like a slide, but will be like a ladder, the stagnation period is a must, so do not give up, just change diet and exercise,

Chapter 8
Weight Loss Questions and Answers

1.Q: Do I need to lose weight?

A:First of all, to see if your weight is within the ideal weight range, the body fatness index BMI (weight/height 2) is calculated according to the definition of obesity defined by the Department of Health.
Normal range: 18.5 ≦ BMI < 24
Overweight: 24 ≦ BMI <27
Mild obesity: 27 ≦ BMI < 30
Moderate obesity: 30 ≦ BMI <35
Severe obesity: BMI ≧35

2.Q: physical weakness, edema, how to lose weight?

A: People with weak constitutions are also weaker than the heart. They are not suitable for a lot of exercise. The more you move, the more you will become tired. If you diet again, you will become fatter. Therefore, those with weak constitutions must eat normally and eat more mineral food. The heart, and to drink plenty of water, it will not be edema.

3.Q: Why do I need to diet to lose weight?

A: Because during weight loss, if you only rely on diet, eat too little, the body's nutrition is not enough, it will easily lead to weakened resistance, cause colds or other diseases, but you can't continue to lose weight.

4. Q: Why do I exercise a lot and sweat a lot?

A: Because the correct weight loss exercise is aerobic exercise, such as walking or climbing stairs, the best effect, a lot of sweating does not mean losing weight. Because we want to reduce body fat is not water,

5. Q: Why lose weight with a low-calorie, balanced diet and exercise?

A: The causes of obesity are caused by improper diet, except for some diseases. When the calorie intake exceeds the body's requirement, the excess calories will be converted into body fat, resulting in overweight and obesity. Weight loss should start with the causes of obesity, reduce caloric intake, but other nutrients can't be reduced, that is, the diet must be low-calorie and balanced, establish a correct diet, in order to maintain weight. In addition to reducing calorie intake, by burning body fat to reduce fat in fat cells, it also helps to lose weight. In addition, exercise can also make muscles stronger and avoid loose skin due to weight loss. Exercise must use its own strength to "move" to be effective. With external instruments oscillating, vibrating, or smearing some oils, ointments, liquids, etc., with the use of push, rub, pinch and other methods, and can't lose weight.

6. Q: What kind of weight loss method is safe?

A: When you lose weight, you must first pay attention to a balanced diet and adequate nutrition. Although weight loss is to avoid excessive calorie intake, various nutrients that the body needs are still indispensable. If you only eat certain types of food, it may cause nutritional deficiencies. Secondly, the speed of weight loss should not be too fast and should not be expected to be as fast as possible. Usually, it is not possible to reduce 5 to 6 kilograms a day or a few days, and if it is reduced in just a few days, it can easily cause other problems. Metabolic dysfunction, harmful to the body, it is recommended to reduce the amount of about 0.5 to 1 kg per week to continue to reduce, will not have adverse effects on the body.

7.Q: Is it possible to eat only vegetables or only meat during weight loss?

A: The calcium content in vegetables and fruits is generally low, and more importantly, it is almost free of fat, which leads to a decrease in the secretion of estrogen in the body, which affects the binding of calcium to bone and prone to osteoporosis. Iron deficiency anemia is more likely to occur in vegetarians! If the food structure is not correct, or calorie intake is reduced, malnutrition, anemia, and hypoproteinemia may result. People who eat only a small amount of vegetables have a much higher chance of suffering from gallstones. Losers who do not eat meat only tend to be depressed. Once they break down, they will lead to overeating and fattening. Excessive fat intake also increases women's chances of developing breast cancer.

8.Q: Can I lose weight by eating only a single food such as apples or vegetables every day?

A: I only eat a single food such as apples or vegetables every day. I mistakenly believe that doing so can reduce intake and fat consumption. Do not eat meat and staple foods, only fruits and vegetables or bananas, although effective weight loss, but the long-term intake of energy is greatly reduced, resulting in malnutrition, anemia, osteoporosis, the probability of occurrence has greatly improved. In fact, a large part of the secret of diet control lies in "quantity." Originally, it was necessary to eat 4 meals, and now it is changed to 2 or 2. If one wants to eat an entire PIZZA, it is now changed to a small piece, so that you can enjoy delicious food. It will not consume too much.

ABOUT THE AUTHOR

The author was born in 1966 and was born in Taiwan. She is engaged in biotechnology and beauty care products and slimming business. She has also been involved in research on traditional Chinese medicine for self-cultivation and Western medicine, and she has also personally experimented with ways to lose weight to find the right one. Ways to lose weight, do a good job of seven revolutions in the brain from food and lifestyle awareness, to a fundamental reconstruction, dieters do not need to diet, do not need a lot of exercise, can easily, healthy, beautiful, happy , Successful weight loss. Will continue to introduce how to spend menopause, prevent heart disease, properly maintain skin and so on.